I0791434

B.R.E.A.T.H.E.

BUILD RESILENCY EVERYDAY AND THINK HEALTH ETERNALLY

BY: JARA CLARK

BREATHE

copyright © by Jara Clark 2020

All rights reserved.

No part of this book may be reproduced or transmitted in any form or by any means without written permission from the author.

Visit us on the web!

www.fitgoddesstribe.com

Printed in the United States of America

ISBN: 9798580608600

Success Stories

I would love to hear your testimony on your experience making these smoothies. Tell me about your success story. Whatever your goal, I'm honored for you to share it with me.

 Email: fitgtribe@gmail.com

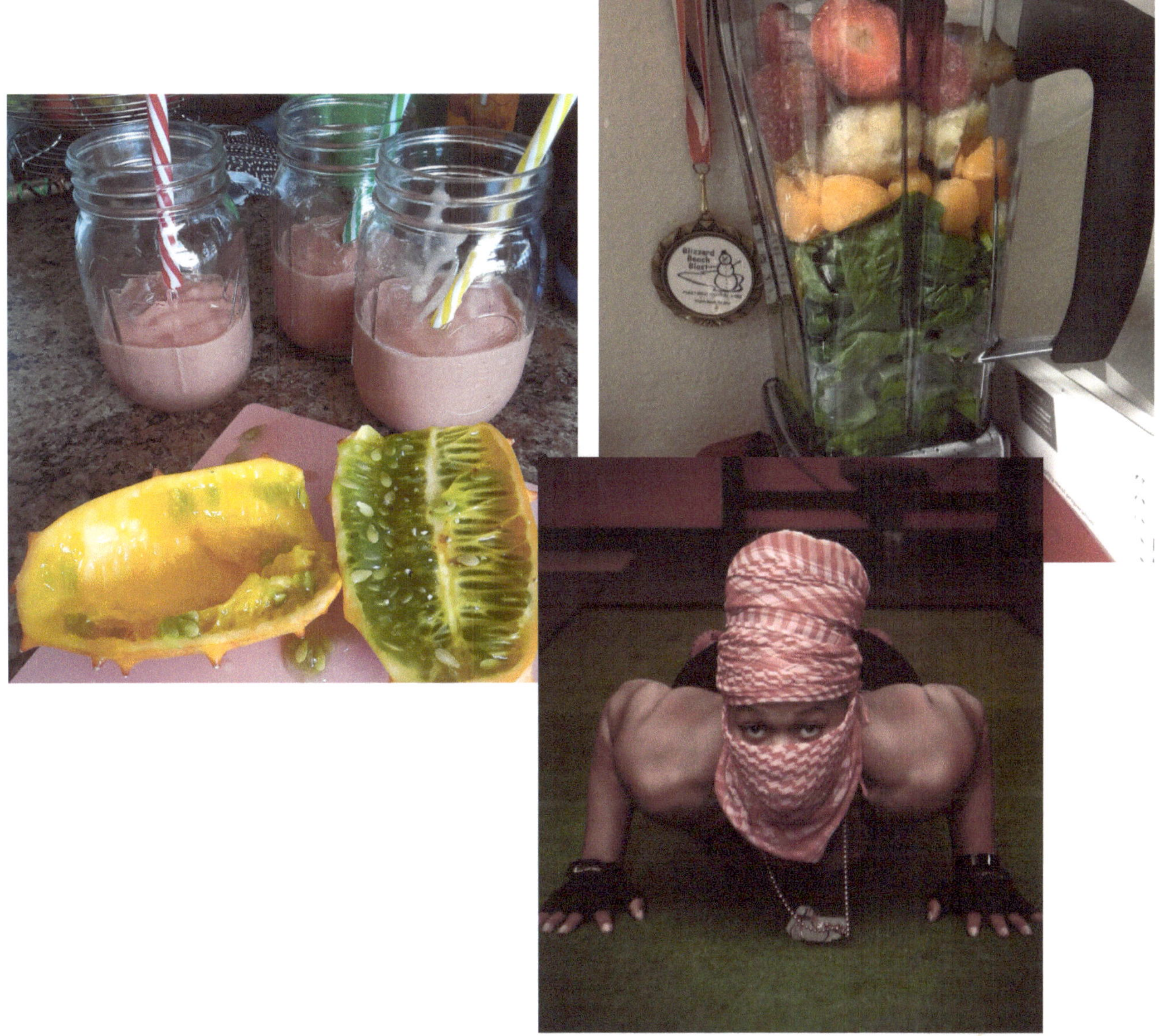

DEDICATION

For Elijah (Eli) and Nasir (Nas) for motivating me to change and
stick to my words to myself.

I am thankful for my mom, Mildred Clark, and brother Kevin Clark.
Despite kidney disease, you both do big things. I aspire to live up to the family
legacy you continue to create. I'm bringing up the rear!
Keep getting better family.

NUTRITION DISCLAIMER

This e-book offers nutritional information and is designed for educational purposes only. You should not rely on this information as a substitute for professional medical advice or treatment. The author is not a medical professional nor claims to have any credentials to support the accuracy of nutritional benefits within these pages. Do not disregard, avoid, or delay obtaining medical or health-related advice from your health-care professional because of something you may have read in this book. The use of any information provided in this book is at the sole choice and risk of the reader.

If you choose to use this information without the prior consent of your physician, you are agreeing to accept full responsibility for your decisions and agreeing to hold harmless Fit Goddess LLC. or its agents, employees, contractors and any affiliated companies from any liability with respect to injury or illness to you connected with your use of the information contained within this book.

CONTENTS

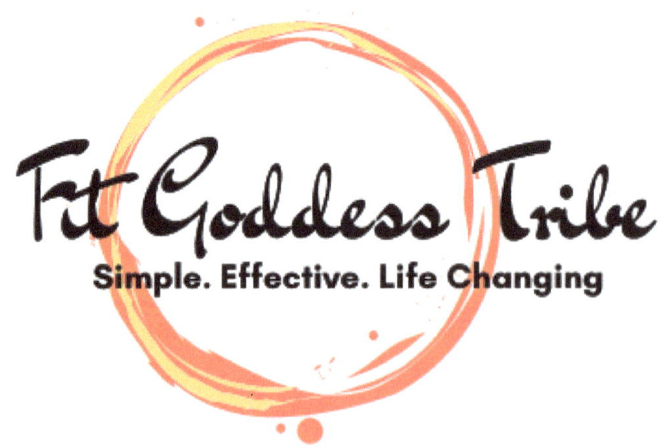

Drink Your Way to Healthy

31 DAYS TO A HEALTHIER YOU

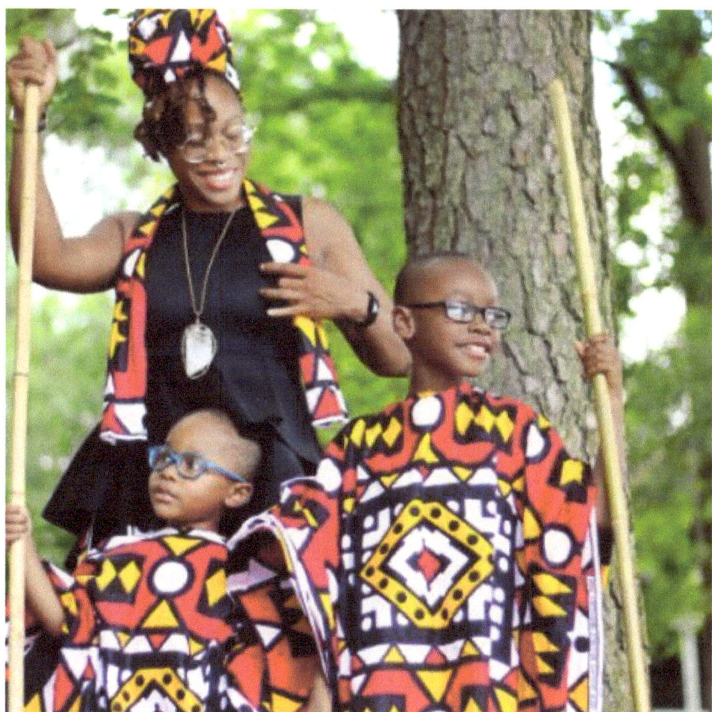

Photo: Dominant Photography

How do we make good healthy food in a simple and delicious way? Nutritious smoothies of course. As a busy mom of two, fitness instructor, and overall active person that is always on the go, smoothies have been my go to food source to get my daily nutrients. These smoothies were originally created for my family and me to make us feel fuller, longer. When I realized they also caused me to have the energy to keep up with two active boys while staying hydrated and getting my daily intake of important vitamins, they became a regular addition to our health journey. Now, I'm happy to offer my family recipes to you!

To some, this may just be a book of delicious drinks to quench the hunger and delight the palate. However, in these pages, there is so much more. The intent of this book is to help you lead the healthy lifestyle you desire and deserve. When used properly this book will give you variety in your diet, confidence in food choices, and more confidence overall. Depending on your goals you can use these drinks as a detox, meal replacements, meal supplements, and even meal enhancers. When detoxing, you are cleansing and refreshing the body. In a way, you are setting it back to "factory default". Cleansing your body strips it of everything causing you to take steps to replenish the body. Not with these smoothies! These recipes work to cleanse and are packed with nutrients and vitamins that replenish the body simultaneously. With these special recipes, I have designed you don't have to take anything additional because the smoothies are packed with the vitamins you need and the flavor you want. You are your greatest priority today and every day. TODAY is a new day and what we do today matters most. Dive in and embrace your new healthy journey. Love yourself back to health.

BUILD

Old Faithful
FIT GODDESS

WHEN ALL ELSE FAILS, GO FOR BERRIES AND BANANAS

There is beauty in simplicity, and this recipe is simply beautiful. If you are looking to start your journey and just need the basics to start towards a healthy lifestyle, Old Faithful is the way to go. Most families usually have these ingredients readily available. We call it Old Faithful because it is the one recipe that's always there, filling and delicious. No skepticism here. Just good deliciousness straight from blender to belly.

You will need

- 2 cup strawberries (fresh or frozen)
- 1 cup bananas (fresh or frozen)
- 8-16 oz. non-dairy milk (almond, cashew, oat, rice, hemp)
- 8-16 oz. juice (coconut water)
- Honey (to taste)

Optional Ingredients

- Plant protein
- Superfood powder mix
- Wheatgrass
- Maca

To Make

Add all ingredients to the blender. Be sure to add the powdered and liquid ingredients last to minimize the mess and maximize your blender's ability. Blend until smooth. Add more liquid for a thinner smoothie, less for a thicker smoothie.

Notes

Tired of smoothies in a cup? Blend this mixture thick and serve in a bowl. Top with your favorite berries, nuts, seeds, whip cream, etc. Fresh berries have more juice and will need less liquid. Make it a family event and locate your nearest farm for some good berry picking, then freeze your harvest and use it as needed.

Living Life Like It's Golden

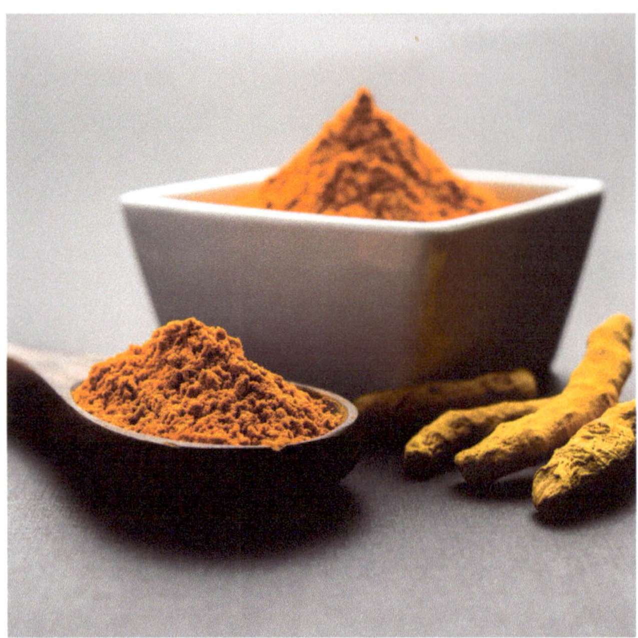

Turmeric is a beautiful simple spice that can enhance your life and make it feel GOLDEN, inside and out. Ever need a bit of sunshine in a cup, this is it. Enhance your shine from the inside out.

You will need

- 1 ½ cup strawberries
- ½ cup cherries
- ½ cup blueberries
- 1-2 Tbsp. Golden Milk Powder
- 2 Tbsp. flaxseed
- 1 scoop superfood blend
- 8-16 oz. liquid (juice, water, or coconut water)

Optional Ingredients

- Plant based protein powder
- Toppings: honey roasted pecans, walnuts, non-dairy whipped topping

To Make

Add all ingredients to the blender. Be sure to add the powdered and liquid ingredients last to minimize the mess and maximize your blender's ability. Blend until smooth. Add more liquid for a thinner smoothie, less for a thicker smoothie.

Notes

Spice up your life! Turmeric blends well with other spices like cinnamon, and cloves. You can add them for an additional flavor. This smoothie is a good bedtime drink for a calming effect. Turmeric decreases inflammation. Using a superfood blend gives you vitamins B6, B12, Thiamin, Niacin, and Riboflavin and includes broccoli vitamin E, vitamin C, tomatoes, vitamin A, as well as vegan protein from pea, hemp, and quinoa. Preferred blends by Better Body Foods.

Sweet Red & Green

It is all about the green and red, life-giving colors. We are less likely to choose certain foods because of their overt bitterness like raspberries. However, that bitterness brightens the naturally sweet flavors of the apples, kale, and strawberries and makes all of the ingredients sweeter. Like life, we need a bit of bitterness to really enjoy the sweet.

You will need

- ½ cup kale
- ¼ cup raspberries
- ½ green apple (cored)
- 1 cup strawberries
- 2 Tbsp. honey
- 8-16 oz. liquid (apple juice or coconut water)

Optional Ingredients

- Plant protein
- Flaxseed
- Moringa powder

To Make

Add all ingredients to the blender. Be sure to add the powdered and liquid ingredients last to minimize the mess and maximize your blender's ability. Blend until smooth. Add more liquid for a thinner smoothie, less for a thicker smoothie.

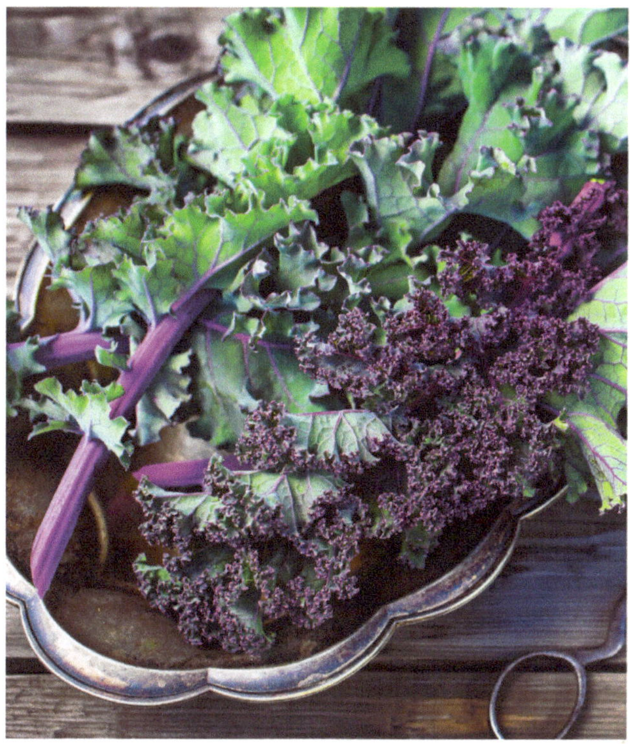

Notes

We use moringa because it is one of the most nutrient-dense plants on this earth. Being more nutritious than kale it boasts 2x more protein, 4x more iron, 3x more calcium, and 2.5x more fiber. Red Delicious isn't the only type of red apple. Each apple bears a different flavor palate. Take the liberty and diversify your apple choices for a different experience each time! Apple picking is an amazing fall activity, make the adventure the prelude to the smoothie for a farm to table experience.

Purple Potion

MY FAVORITE ROYAL BREW

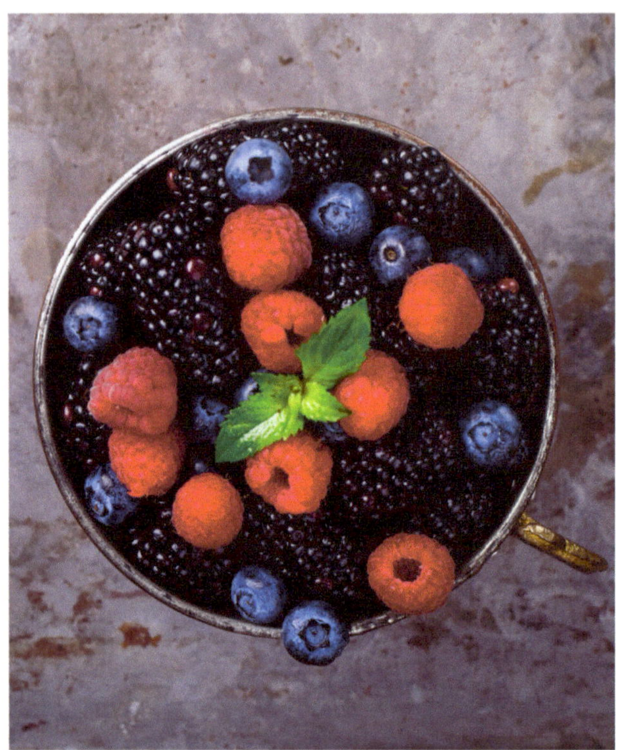

Immunity Booster. Our ability to fight off dis-ease is largely attributed to our immune system. Dis-ease is when the body or mind is in a state of unease, which means it is not functioning properly. A body or mind that does not function properly will eventually manifest disease. Why not give it a BOOST daily!

You will need

- ½ cup red raspberries
- 1 cup strawberries
- ½ cup blackberries
- ½ cup blueberries
- 4-8 oz. pomegranate juice
- Add a4-8 oz. elderberry juice
- 2-4 Tbsp. honey or to taste

Optional Ingredients

- Protein powder
- Superfood Blend
- Wheat Grass
- Flaxseed
- Sea Moss

To Make

Add all ingredients to the blender. Be sure to add the powdered and liquid ingredients last to minimize the mess and maximize your blender's ability. Blend until smooth. Add more liquid for a thinner smoothie, less for a thicker smoothie.

Notes

Berries are some of the healthiest foods you can eat, as they are low in calories but high in fiber, vitamin C, and antioxidants. Many berries have proven benefits for heart health. These include lowering blood pressure and cholesterol while reducing oxidative stress. Elderberries are packed with antioxidants and vitamins that boost your immune system. They help with inflammation, lessen stress. Elderberry is recommended to help prevent and ease cold and flu symptoms.

Rainbow Peach Dragon

BITE THE PEACH BUT DON'T BURN THE FRUIT

Sweet, juicy, and delicious with all the fire and power of the dragon. The sweetest in the dragon family, filled with a variety of delectable fruits.

You will need

- ½ cup peaches
- ¼ cup pineapple
- ½ cup blueberries
- 1 cup strawberries
- ¼ cup dragon fruit
- ¼ cup avocado
- 1 scoop superfood powder
- 1-2 Tbsp. flaxseed

Optional Ingredients

- Plant based protein powder
- Whey isolate protein

To Make

Add all ingredients to the blender. Be sure to add the powdered and liquid ingredients last to minimize the mess and maximize your blender's ability. Blend until smooth. Add more liquid for a thinner smoothie, less for a thicker smoothie.

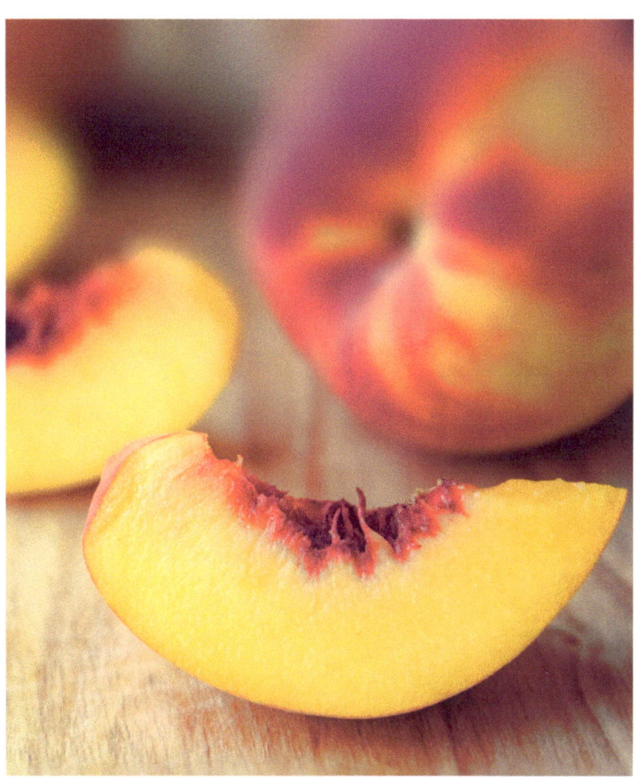

Notes

Peaches are high in fiber, vitamins, and minerals with beneficial plant compounds like antioxidants. These help aid in protecting your body from aging and disease. Peaches are also known to help lower your immune system's response to allergens, thus reducing allergy symptoms. Just like we were told in grade school fruits are sources of many essential nutrients. Most notably potassium, dietary fiber, vitamin C, and folate (folic acid). Diets rich in potassium may help to maintain healthy blood pressure.

Cocoa Berry Cream

THE BLACKER THE BERRY THEY SAY

A few of our favorite things. Each rich in vitamins, antioxidants, potassium, and most importantly flavor. Whoever said healthy had to taste bad must have missed the memo.

You will need

- 1 ½ cup strawberries
- ½ cup peaches
- ½ cup bananas
- ½ cup avocados
- 1 scoop cocoa or chocolate protein powder

Seasonings

- ¼ tsp. cinnamon
- A pinch of nutmeg and clove

To Make

Add all ingredients to the blender. Be sure to add the powdered and liquid ingredients last to minimize the mess and maximize your blender's ability. Blend until smooth. Add more liquid for a thinner smoothie, less for a thicker smoothie.

Notes

Who would have thought chocolate would be so beneficial. Unprocessed cocoa can improve blood flow, reduce cholesterol, and risk of heart attack, heart failure, and stroke. Cocoa positively affects mood and symptoms of depression by reducing stress levels. It also promotes calmness, contentment, and overall psychological well-being.

Straight Strawberry

When we say simple and effective, we really mean it. It doesn't get much simpler than this. Love, passion, and heart health are all words associated with the color RED and our favorite berry. Add this super fruit to your diet.

You will need

- 2-3 cups of frozen strawberries
- 8-16 oz. liquid (juice, milk, or water)
- 2-3 Tbsp. honey

Optional Ingredients

- Sea Moss

To Make

Add all ingredients to the blender. Be sure to add the powdered and liquid ingredients last to minimize the mess and maximize your blender's ability. Blend until smooth. Add more liquid for a thinner smoothie, less for a thicker smoothie.

Notes

Strawberries are an excellent source of vitamin C. Vitamin C is a well-known immunity booster. Strawberries are also a powerful and fast working antioxidant. Antioxidants protect the body from free radicals that may produce disease. We need strong antioxidants to maintain our internal health.

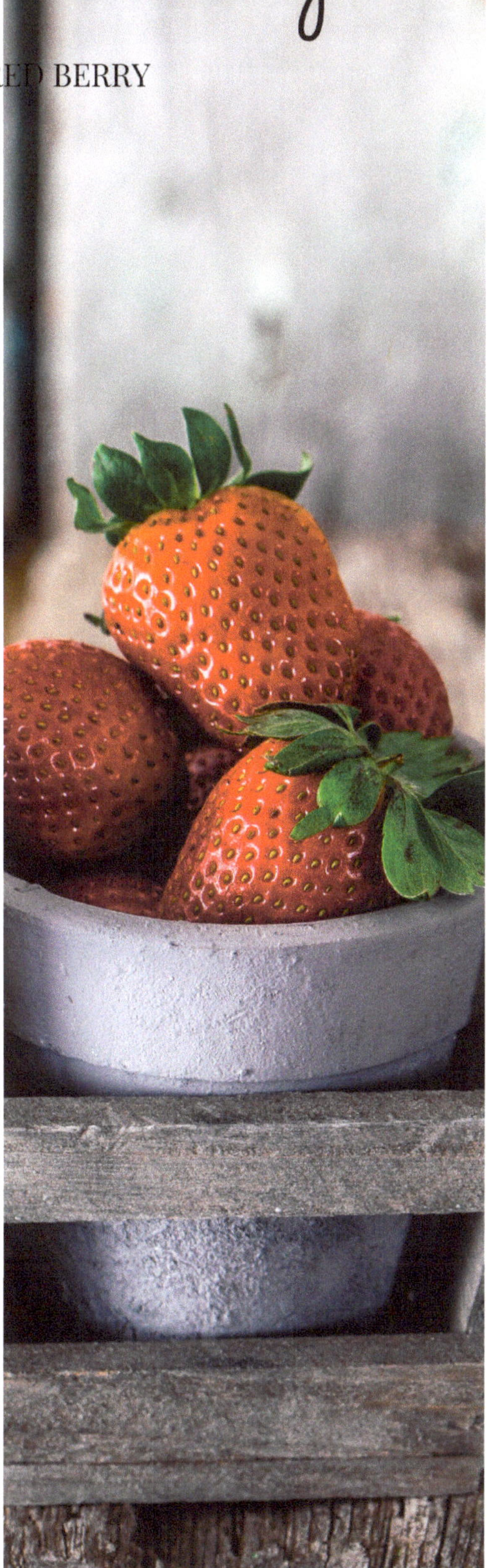

RESILIENCY

Strawberries and Cream
FIT GODDESS

THE PERFECT TEAM

One of the ultimate sweet treats turned healthy. Just the right dose of naturally sweet, sinfully smooth, and best of all GOOD for you!

You will need

- 2 cups strawberries
- 1 cup bananas
- ½ cup non-dairy yogurt
- 8-16 oz. non-dairy milk
- 2 Tbsp. flaxseed
- 2 Tbsp. honey

Optional Ingredients

- Vanilla plant based protein powder

To Make

Add all ingredients to the blender. Be sure to add the powdered and liquid ingredients last to minimize the mess and maximize your blender's ability. Blend until smooth. Add more liquid for a thinner smoothie, less for a thicker smoothie.

Notes

Flaxseed supports cardiovascular health and contains 3g of ALAOMEGA 3. Strawberries can be substituted with other fruits (peaches, raspberries, blueberries, blackberries) Turn it into a " Green Smoothie" by adding greens of your choice. Kale is great but bitter, remember to add a bit more sweet fruit or honey to sweeten or use spinach.

Snickerdoodle Green

CINNAMON GOODNESS

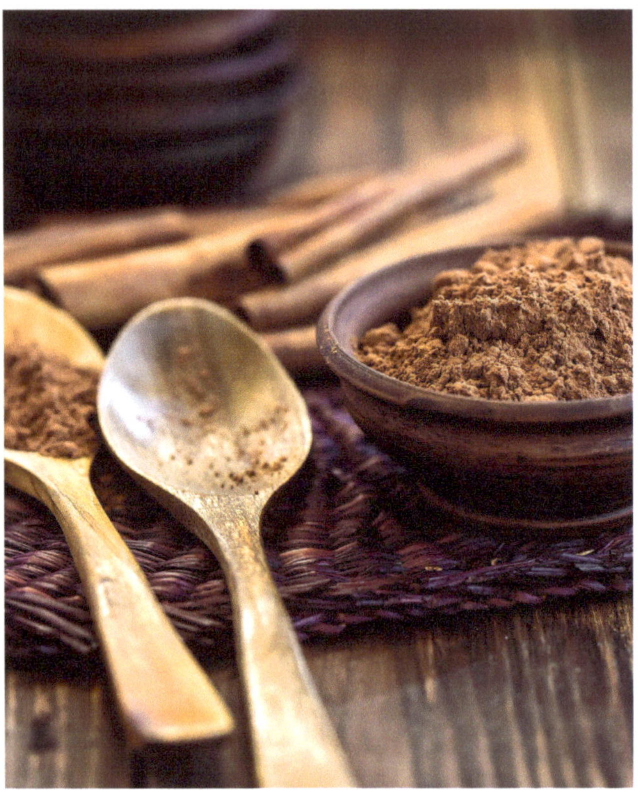

Cookies in a cup, this holiday treat turns green. When what you want most is sweet, make it green and call it good. Healthy is abundantly sweet, much like this smoothie. Use it to boost your health daily!

You will need

- 2 cups of spinach
- 2 frozen bananas
- 1 small avocado
- 1½ cup unsweetened almond milk
- 1 tsp. vanilla
- ½ tsp. cinnamon

Optional Ingredients

- Sea Moss
- Wheat Grass

Notes

Wheatgrass enhances the function of your immune system. This can help ward off infection and disease. Much like a well-maintained machine, not only will you feel better when your immune system is performing well, it only stands to increase as you work towards higher levels of health.

To Make

Add all ingredients to the blender. Be sure to add the powdered and liquid ingredients last to minimize the mess and maximize your blender's ability. Blend until smooth. Add more liquid for a thinner smoothie, less for a thicker smoothie.

Blueberry Cobbler

You don't have to necessarily give up the things you enjoy. Just rethink how to enjoy them. This smoothie having you craving this sweet treat the normally hot, in a new way!

You will need

- 1 cup frozen blueberries
- 1 banana fresh or frozen
- ¾ cup milk
- 1 Tbsp. honey
- 1 Tbsp. golden flaxseed
- ½ tsp. fresh-squeezed lemon juice
- ¾ tsp. cinnamon
- Pinch of nutmeg

Optional Ingredients

- Non-diary whipped topping
- Honey roasted pecans, walnuts
- Crush cashews

To Make

Add all ingredients to the blender. Be sure to add the powdered and liquid ingredients last to minimize the mess and maximize your blender's ability. Blend until smooth. Add more liquid for a thinner smoothie, less for a thicker smoothie.

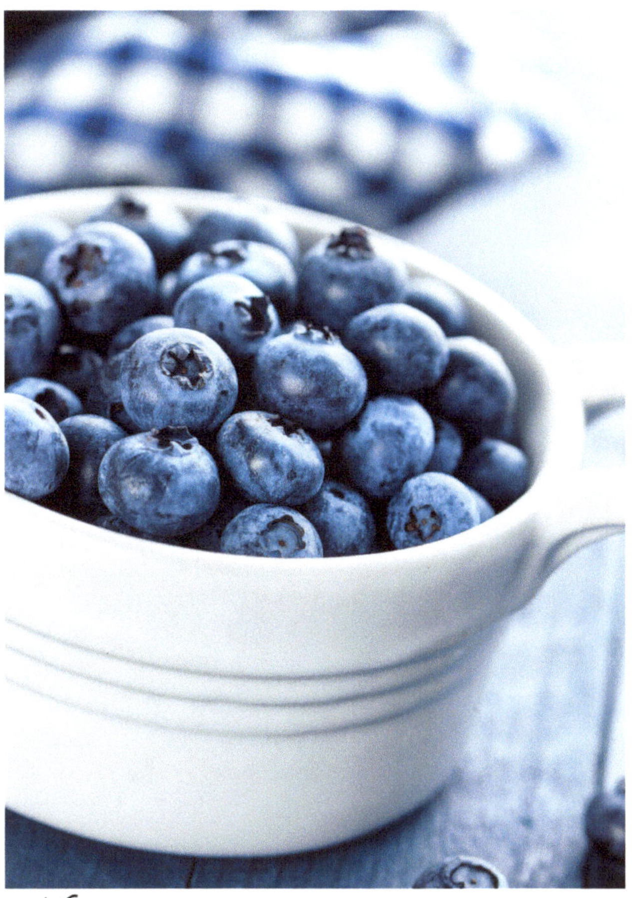

Notes

This smoothie allows us to show how powerful the brain is. It is all about the choice! This smoothie will have you believing you are having the most delicious cobbler with all the fat yet, in reality, you are not losing the taste you are gaining the added benefits of healthier choices. Blueberries can be switched out for peaches or any other "pie" filling. Ex. apple, peaches, strawberries.

Sunrise

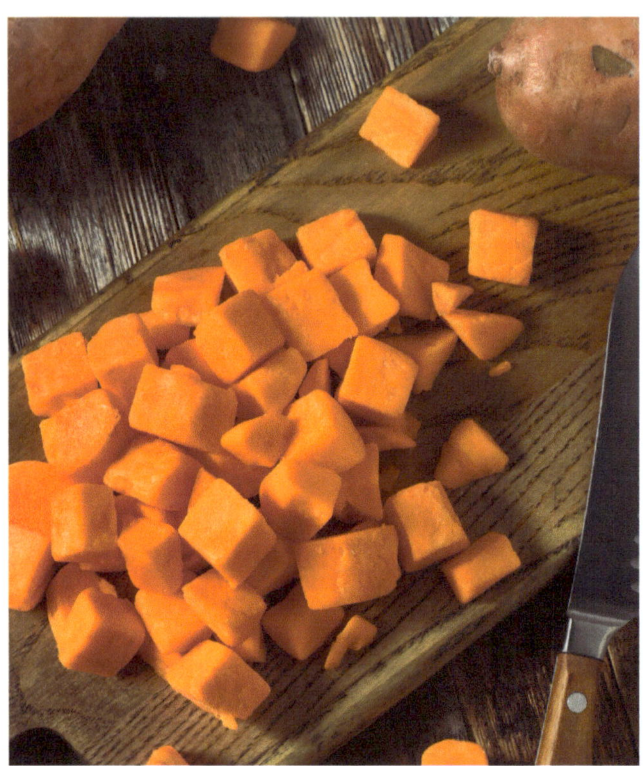

The best way to kick start a gloomy day is with a bit of internal sunshine. Take 10 minutes and brighten your day by filling your cup with a bit of sunrise.

You will need

- 1 cup mandarin orange
- 1 banana
- ½ cup pineapple
- ½ mango
- ¼ sweet potato

Optional Ingredients

- Sea Moss

Notes

Sweet potatoes are a superfood that promotes gut health. They are a starchy root vegetable, rich in fiber, vitamins, and minerals. They're also high in antioxidants that protect your body from free radical damage and chronic disease.

To Make

Add all ingredients to the blender. Be sure to add the powdered and liquid ingredients last to minimize the mess and maximize your blender's ability. Blend until smooth. Add more liquid for a thinner smoothie, less for a thicker smoothie.

Berry Red Dragon

RETURN OF THE DRAGON

All the best fruits and berries to get the blood pumping and infused with powerful nutrients. Nourish yourself with the bounty of the berries.

You will need

- 1 cup strawberries
- 1 banana
- ½ red cherries
- ½ cup dragon fruit
- ¼ cranberries
- 2-4 Tbsp. honey
- 8-16 oz. juice or coconut water

Optional Ingredients

- Sea Moss
- Wheat Grass (add a bit more honey, as wheat grass can be bitter)

To Make

Add all ingredients to the blender. Be sure to add the powdered and liquid ingredients last to minimize the mess and maximize your blender's ability. Blend until smooth. Add more liquid for a thinner smoothie, less for a thicker smoothie.

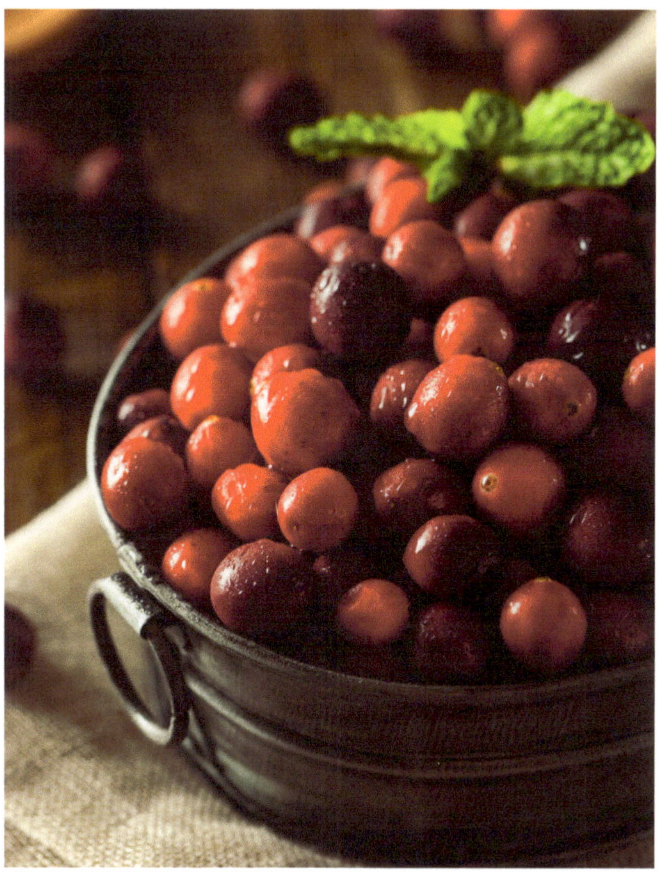

Notes

Cranberries are known for lowering the risk of urinary tract infections (UTI), they also aid in the prevention of certain types of cancer, improved immune function, and decreased blood pressure. Cherries are full of antioxidants, fiber, calcium, and vitamin C that help protect against chronic diseases and boost your recovery after exercise.

Sweet Green & Gold

Behold the deliciousness that is the Sweet Green & Gold. Your body will feel as rich as if you were coating your insides with the beauty of green and the richness of gold. This drink is a thirst quencher for the royals.

You will need

- 1 cup mango
- 1 banana
- ½ cup red apple
- ½ pineapple
- ½ cup spinach
- 2-4 Tbsp. honey
- 8 oz. juice or coconut water

Optional Ingredients

- Wheatgrass
- Sea moss
- Superfood blend
- Plant based protein powder

To Make

Add all ingredients to the blender. Be sure to add the powdered and liquid ingredients last to minimize the mess and maximize your blender's ability. Blend until smooth. Add more liquid for a thinner smoothie, less for a thicker smoothie.

Notes

Mango is low in calories yet high in nutrients- particularly vitamin C, which aids immunity, iron absorption and growth, and repair. It is also loaded with fibrous content, it boosts the digestive function and burns unwanted calories from the body.

How She Get That Energy

Have you ever had a day where you just needed a little bit more? We have those moments, where we would prefer to do nothing but everything needs to get done. This no-fuss, quick drink will give you a much-needed jump start to get you through your day.

You will need

- 3-4 matcha green tea cubes
- 1 banana
- 1 cup mango
- ¼ pineapple
- 2-4 Tbsp. honey
- 8 oz juice or coconut water

To Make

Add all ingredients to the blender. Be sure to add the powdered and liquid ingredients last to minimize the mess and maximize your blender's ability. Blend until smooth. Add more liquid for a thinner smoothie, less for a thicker smoothie.

Notes

Matcha improves several aspects of brain function including attention, memory, and reaction time. Matcha increases metabolism and fat burning, both of which may aid in weight loss.

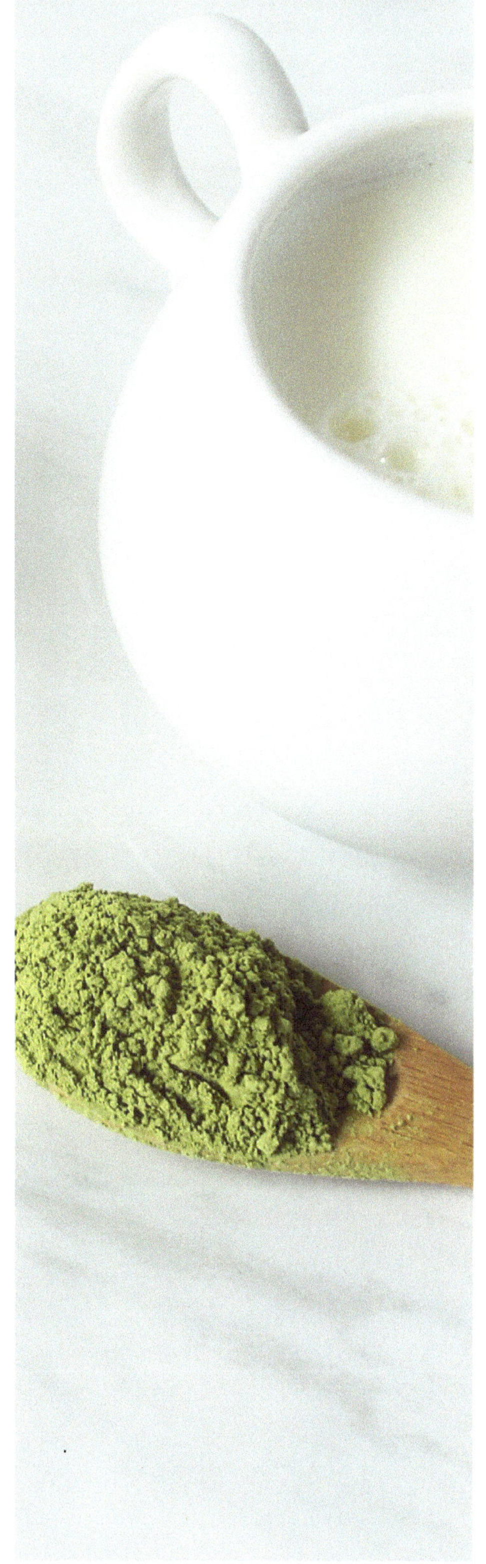

THINK HEALTH

Fat Red Dragon
FIT GODDESS

THE GOOD KIND OF FAT

Like in life, too much of anything is bad. Likewise, not enough of something can be EQUALLY as bad. The body needs fat, just in small healthy doses. This dragon is a balance of heart-healthy fats and a delicious immune boost.

You will need

- ¼ cup dragon fruit
- ¼ cup peaches
- ¼ cup strawberries
- ¼ cup bananas
- ½ cup avocadoes
- ¼ tsp. ginger
- 1 scoop superfood blend protein powder
- 1 scoop plant protein
- 1-2 Tbsp. flaxseed
- 8-16 oz. liquid (coconut water, juice, or water)

To Make

Add all ingredients to the blender. Be sure to add the powdered and liquid ingredients last to minimize the mess and maximize your blender's ability. Blend until smooth. Add more liquid for a thinner smoothie, less for a thicker smoothie.

Notes

Coconuts are an all-natural way to hydrate, reduce sodium. As a bonus, they also add potassium to diets. Avocados are "good" fat. They are a great source of vitamins C, E, K, and B-6 plus riboflavin, niacin, folate, pantothenic acid, magnesium, and potassium.

Lavender Creme

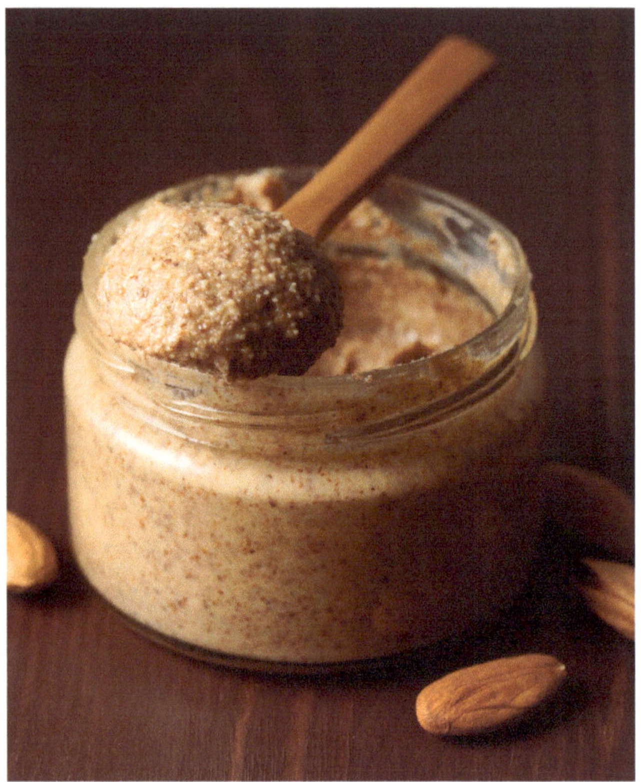

The natural dark purple hue of blueberries, mixed with the silky smooth white from the creamy coconut milk, blends to a beautiful lavender color. The color alone is soothing. This drink is packed with protein and iron with a smooth taste. Just what the body needs for constant regeneration.

You will need

- 2 cups blueberries
- 1 banana
- 1 scoop protein powder
- 2-3 Tbsp. almond butter
- 2 Tbsp. honey
- 8 oz. coconut milk

Optional Ingredients

- Sea moss
- ¼ tsp. ground cloves powder

Notes

Almond butter is an excellent way to access the health benefits of almonds all year long. Almond butter is a great source of vitamin E, magnesium, copper, vitamin B2 (riboflavin), and phosphorus. It is a great source of monounsaturated fat, the good kind of fat you need in your diet. Almond butter adds protein, and fiber which are essential for heart health.

To Make

Add all ingredients to the blender. Be sure to add the powdered and liquid ingredients last to minimize the mess and maximize your blender's ability. Blend until smooth. Add more liquid for a thinner smoothie, less for a thicker smoothie.

Pumpkin Pie Bliss

SATISFY THAT PUMPKIN CRAVING

This Fall drink can be made anytime you want as a sweet treat or dessert. Our favorite part of family dinner, this has all the fun and flavor of homemade pie and the added bonus of healthy ingredients. Indulge in this delectable and healthy alternative.

You will need

- ½ cup canned pumpkin or ½ cooked sweet potatoes
- ¾ tsp. cinnamon
- ½ tsp. nutmeg
- ½ tsp. pumpkin pie spice
- 1 ½ - 2 cups coconut or almond milk
- 1 scoop vanilla protein powder
- 1 Tbsp. flaxseed
- 2 Tbsp. honey
- 6 ice cubes (to make more creamy freeze 6 cubes of milk ahead of time)

Toppings

- 2 Tbsp. honey roasted pecans
- Whip Cream

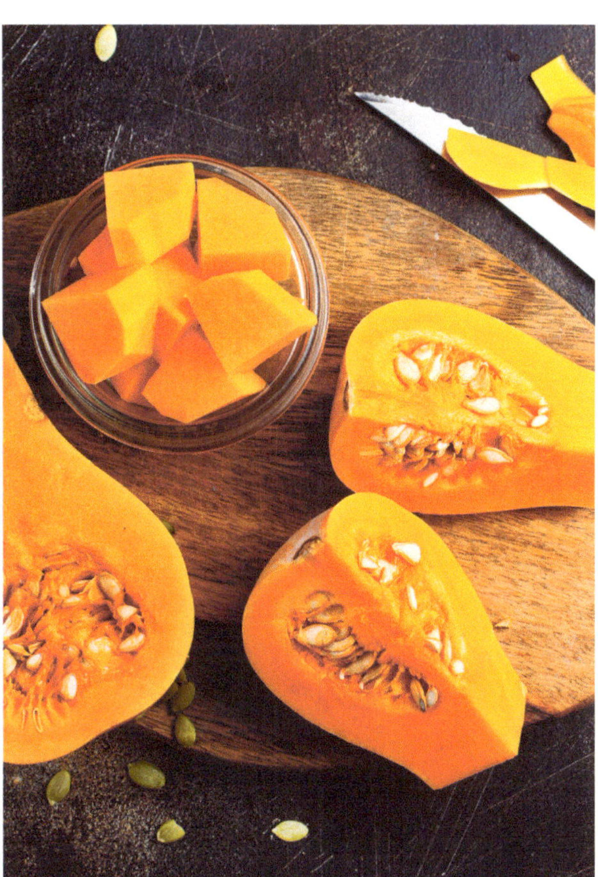

To Make

Add all ingredients to the blender. Be sure to add the powdered and liquid ingredients last to minimize the mess and maximize your blender's ability. Blend until smooth. Add more liquid for a thinner smoothie, less for a thicker smoothie.

Notes

Pumpkin is high in vitamins and minerals while being low in calories. It is also a great source of beta-carotene, which helps you see better. Flaxseed is a plant-based food that provides healthful fat, antioxidants, and fiber. The antioxidants in honey have been linked to beneficial effects on heart health, including increased blood flow to your heart and a reduced risk of blood clot formation.

Watermelon & Mint Refresher

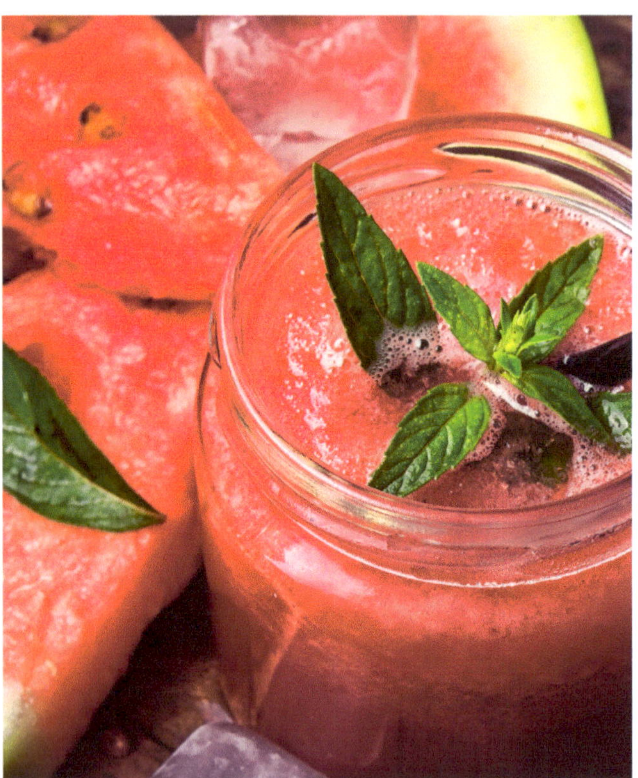

Watermelon is a great way to get that extra boost of water and sweetness when the last thing you may want is water. Mint is not just a breath freshener but adds flavor.

You will need

- 2 cups frozen watermelon
- 1½ frozen strawberries
- 5-10 mint leaves
- 2-4 Tbsp. honey
- 8 oz. coconut water or juice

Optional Ingredients

- Sea moss

Notes

Watermelon is full of vitamins A and C, which support immune function and skin health. Watermelon helps lower blood pressure and improve circulation while reducing muscle soreness. The aroma of peppermint oil improves memory and alertness. Mint oil can speed up how quickly food moves through the stomach, relieving digestive symptoms associated with indigestion.

To Make

Add all ingredients to the blender. Be sure to add the powdered and liquid ingredients last to minimize the mess and maximize your blender's ability. Blend until smooth. Add more liquid for a thinner smoothie, less for a thicker smoothie.

Avocado

FAT AND GREEN

Avocado is a mean green fatty machine. Far from mediocre, this smoothie is packed with nutrients, fats, and enzymes this delicious smoothie is a delightful treat.

You will need

- ½ cup spinach
- ½ cup avocado
- 1 cup juice or coconut water
- 1 cup pineapple
- 2 tsp lemon juice
- ¼ tsp ground ginger

Optional Ingredients

- Sea moss
- Wheatgrass
- Plant based protein

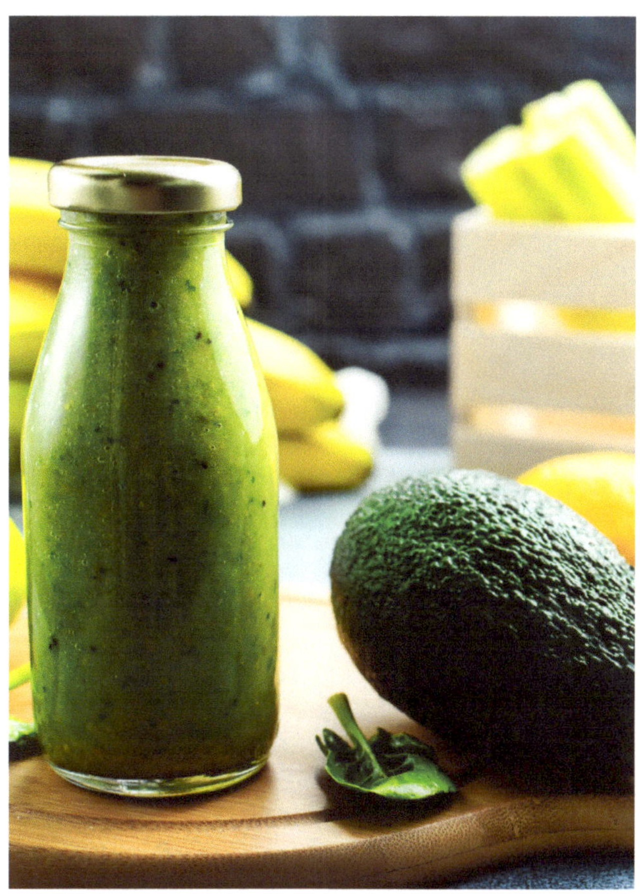

To Make

Add all ingredients to the blender. Be sure to add the powdered and liquid ingredients last to minimize the mess and maximize your blender's ability. Blend until smooth. Add more liquid for a thinner smoothie, less for a thicker smoothie.

Notes

Avocados are loaded with healthy fat that keeps you feeling fuller longer so you will be less likely to snack. Avocados contain potassium, dietary fiber, and fats, not to mention vitamins A, E, K, and B6, which contribute to the health of your heart, blood, and vision.

Apple Pie

WHY NOT PIE!

Apple pies are very delicious but very labor intensive. That doesn't mean we don't deserve this decadent dessert smoothie. All the pleasure of pie with less calories.

You will need

- 2-3 apples
- 1-1 ½ tsp. cinnamon
- 2 tsp. honey
- ¾ cup honey
- ¼ cup rolled oats
- 1 teaspoon vanilla extract
- ⅛-¼ ground nutmeg

Optional Ingredients

- Non-dairy whipped topped
- Honey roasted pecans or walnuts

To Make

Add all ingredients to the blender. Be sure to add the powdered and liquid ingredients last to minimize the mess and maximize your blender's ability. Blend until smooth. Add more liquid for a thinner smoothie, less for a thicker smoothie.

Notes

Apples aid in weight loss, are filling, and high in fiber. They are anti-inflammatory that helps regulate immune responses and protect against asthma. Apples help to lower cholesterol and blood pressure. Make it a family event and locate your nearest farm for some good fruit picking. Freeze your harvest and use it as needed. Apples can be switched out for peaches or any other "pie" filling

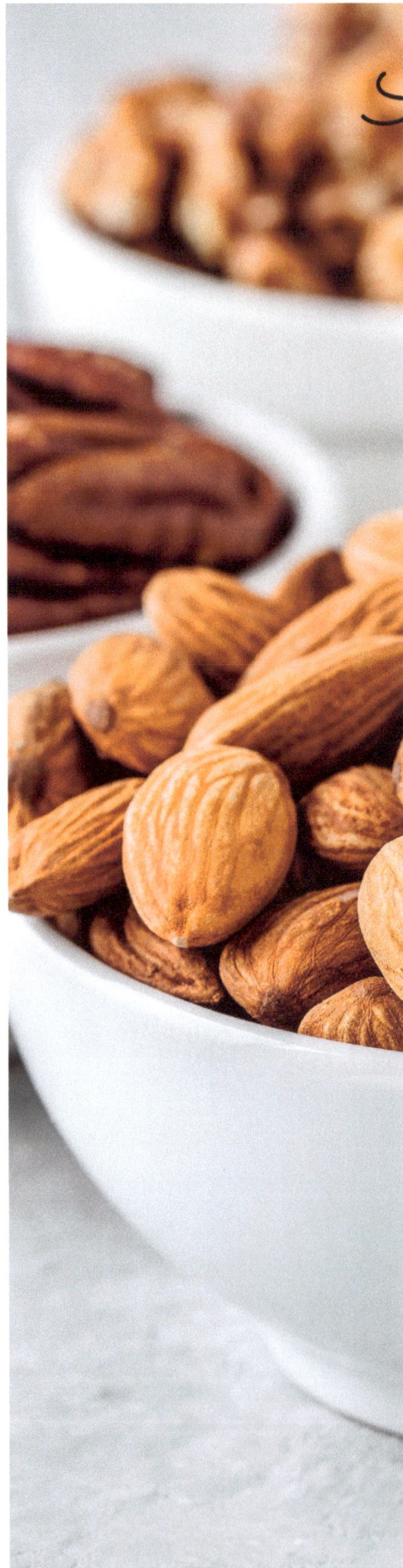

Lean and Green

FIGHTING MACHINE

Your body is a beautiful machine that deserves high-quality fuel. Lean looks different on everyone. Green is the color of life.
Fill your body will the things that will keep it lean and filled with life.

You will need

- 1 ½ cup juice or coconut water
- ½ large avocado
- ½ cup frozen mango
- 1 cup chopped kale
- 1 Tbsp. chia seed
- 2 Tbsp. honey
- 1 Tbsp. flaxseed

Optional Ingredients

- Sea moss
- Wheatgrass
- Plant based protein

To Make

Add all ingredients to the blender. Be sure to add the powdered and liquid ingredients last to minimize the mess and maximize your blender's ability. Blend until smooth. Add more liquid for a thinner smoothie, less for a thicker smoothie.

Notes

Chia seeds are an ancient superfood. It was a mainstay in Aztec and Mayan diets because of its nutritional value. The word "chia" means strength in the Mayan language, and the seeds were known as runner's fuel. This concentrated protein source is also rich in fiber, helping keep the body full and energized for hours.

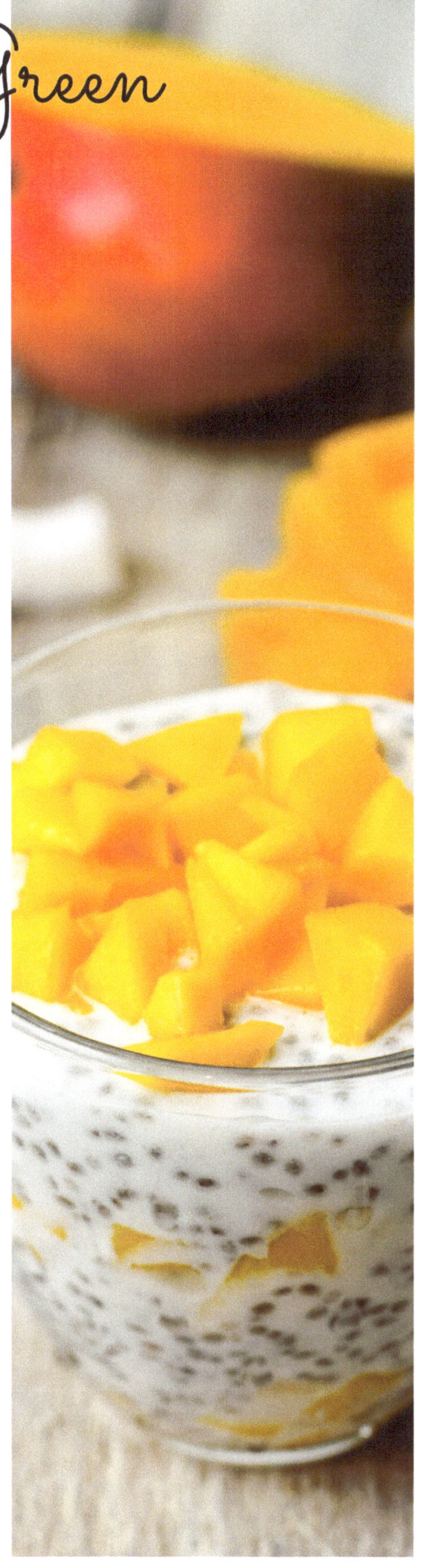

ETERNALLY

Water Dragon
FIT GODDESS

EAT YOUR WATER LIKE A BEAST

Your body is 70% water. This smoothie offers another way to get water to your brain, heart, lungs, muscles, and kidneys. Eat your water through vegetables and fruits.

You will need

- 1 cup dragon fruit
- ¼ cup wheatgrass
- ½ cup watermelon
- ¼ cup kale
- ¼ cup red apples
- ¼ cup mandarin
- 2-4 tablespoons honey
- 8-16 oz. liquid (water, coconut water, or juice)

To Make

Add all ingredients to the blender. Be sure to add the powdered and liquid ingredients last to minimize the mess and maximize your blender's ability. Blend until smooth. Add more liquid for a thinner smoothie, less for a thicker smoothie.

Notes

Water Provides Essential functions that keep us going. Water is a vital nutrient to the life of every cell. It regulates our internal body temperature through sweating. It helps form saliva, a major component in the digestive system. It carries carbohydrates and proteins through our bodies that we metabolize and use as food. Water assists in flushing waste mainly through urination and acts as a shock absorber for the brain, spinal cord, the fetus and it lubricates joints. Water forms saliva, a major component in the digestive system

The Green Tropics

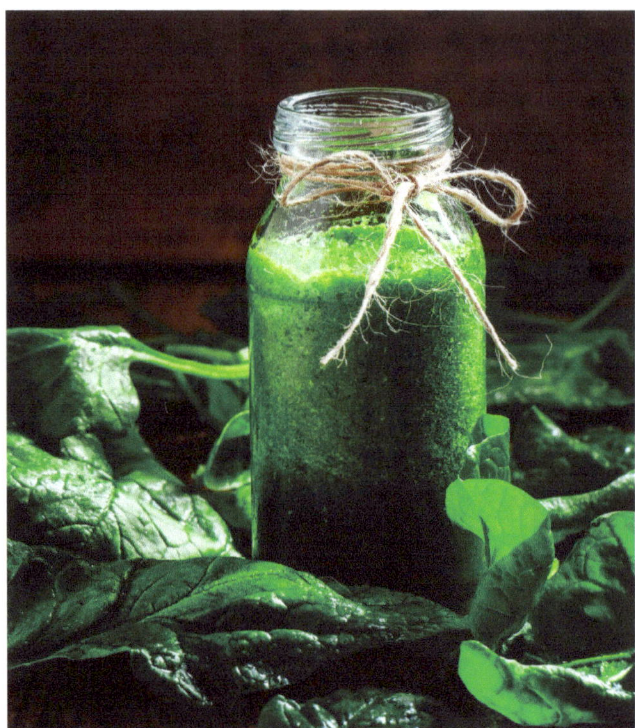

Green goodness from the islands. There's something delightful about the thought of the fruit that comes from the warm weather and pretty blue waters. Now imagine what those beautiful fruits do for your insides.

You will need

- 1-1½ cups coconut water
- 1½ cups tropical fruit blend (pineapple, mango, coconut, strawberries, etc.)
- 1 cup baby spinach
- 2 Tbsp. honey

Optional Ingredients

- Sea moss
- Plant based protein powder

Notes

Spinach is extremely nutrient-rich, promoting eye health, fighting cancer, and regulating blood pressure. Mango is low in calories yet high in nutrients- particularly vitamin C, which aids immunity, iron absorption, growth, and repair. Eating pineapple enhances weight loss and aids in digestion.

To Make

Add all ingredients to the blender. Be sure to add the powdered and liquid ingredients last to minimize the mess and maximize your blender's ability. Blend until smooth. Add more liquid for a thinner smoothie, less for a thicker smoothie.

Berry Muffin

Our favorite now fluffy but still sweet treat. If bread is supposedly bad, this is a sure-fire way to get all the soft and sweet taste and ditch the bread.

You will need

- 1-1½ non-dairy milk
- ½ frozen banana
- 1 cup frozen blueberries
- 2 Tbsp. old fashioned rolled oats
- 2 tablespoons pecans, almonds, or walnuts

Optional Ingredients

- Non-dairy whipped topping
- Plant based protein vanilla flavored.

To Make

Oats are rich in carbs and fiber but also higher in protein and fat than most other grains. Oatmeal helps you lose weight by making you feel more full, slowing down the emptying of the stomach.

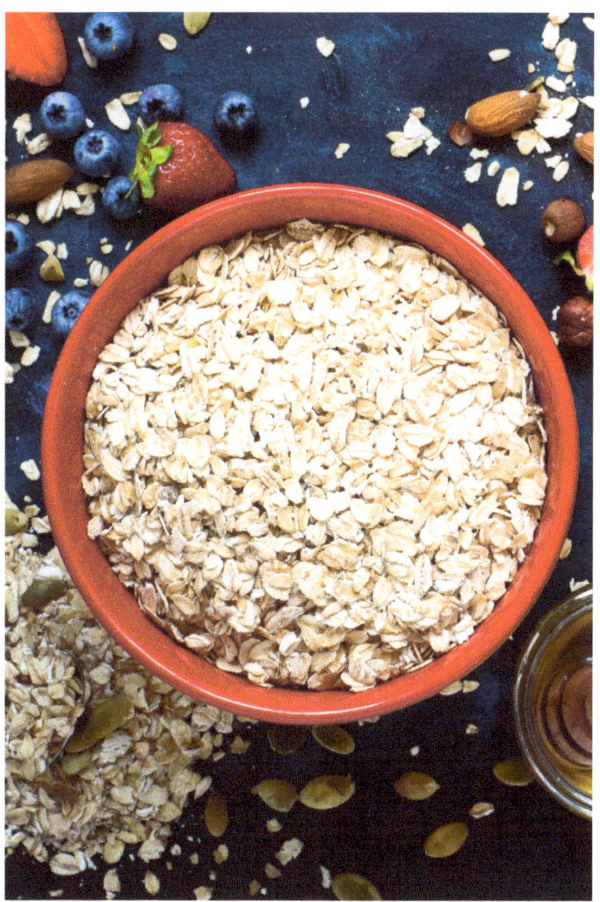

Notes

Add all ingredients to the blender. Be sure to add the powdered and liquid ingredients last to minimize the mess and maximize your blender's ability. Blend until smooth. Add more liquid for a thinner smoothie, less for a thicker smoothie.

Cherries and Chocolate

PLEASE COVER ME

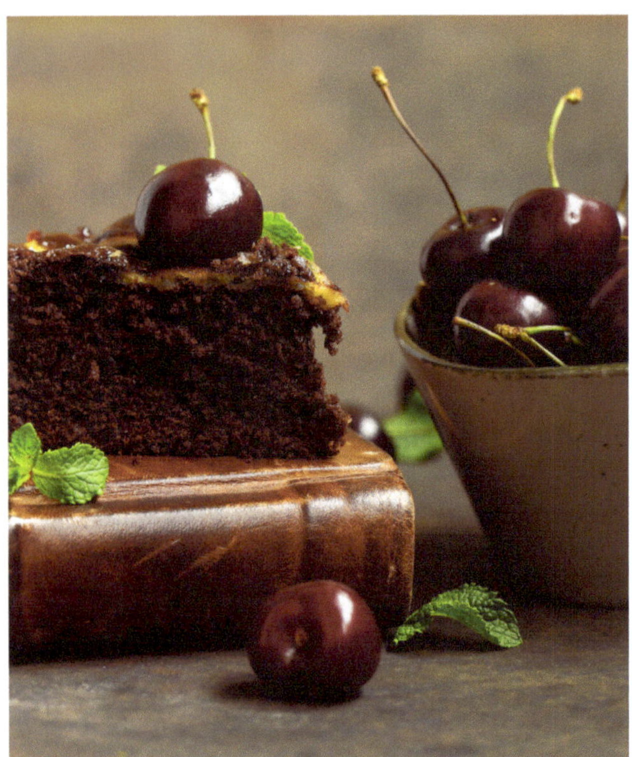

Why wait for Valentine's day to indulge in such sweetness. The antioxidants alone are enough to cause you to rethink your indulgence. No need to sacrifice the sweet, especially with this treat.

You will need

- 1-1½ non-dairy milk
- ½ banana
- 1 cup froze SWEET dark cherries
- 1 cup spinach
- 2 Tbsp. nut butter
- 1 Tbsp. 100% cocoa powder or cacao powder
- 1-2 Tbsp. honey

Notes

Cocoa improves blood flow and reduces cholesterol. Eating up to one serving of chocolate per day may reduce your risk of heart attack, heart failure, and stroke. Cherries are high in antioxidants and anti-inflammatory compounds, which may reduce chronic disease risk and promote overall health.

Optional Ingredients

- Plant based protein powder chocolate flavor

To Make

Add all ingredients to the blender. Be sure to add the powdered and liquid ingredients last to minimize the mess and maximize your blender's ability. Blend until smooth. Add more liquid for a thinner smoothie, less for a thicker smoothie.

Berry Bonanza

BONANZA MEANS BOUNTIFUL

Bonanza is defined as a situation or event that creates a sudden increase in wealth, good fortune, or profits. Imagine what good fortune berries bring for the body. Pair that with the nutrient-packed greens. A bonanza of benefits is what you will receive!

You will need

- 1-1¼ cup non-dairy milk
- ¼ cup vanilla Greek yogurt
- ½ banana
- 1 cup of frozen mixed berries
- 1 cup packed spinach or kale
- 1 Tbsp. ground flaxseed

Optional Ingredients

- Vanilla flavor plant based protein powder

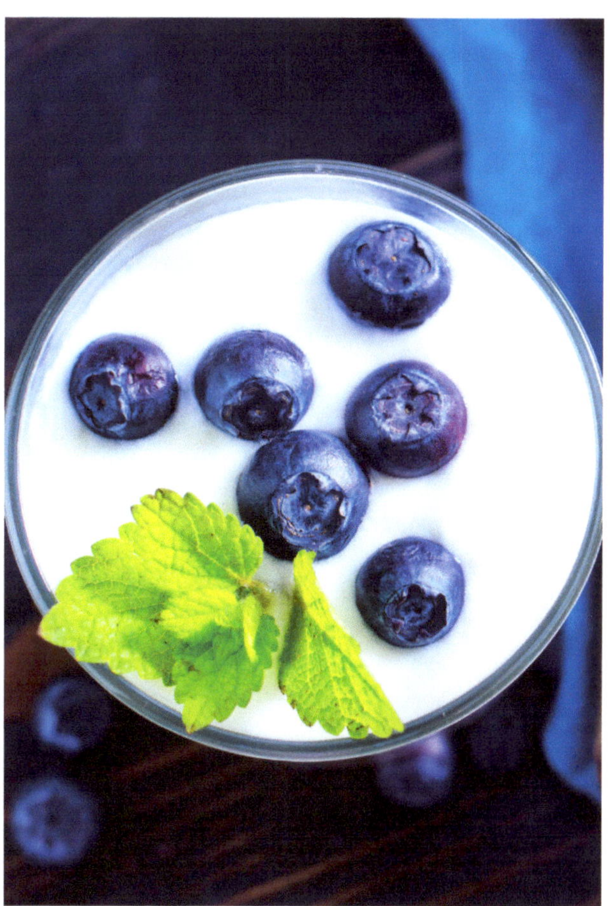

To Make

Add all ingredients to the blender. Be sure to add the powdered and liquid ingredients last to minimize the mess and maximize your blender's ability. Blend until smooth. Add more liquid for a thinner smoothie, less for a thicker smoothie.

Notes

Berries contain fiber which may increase feelings of fullness as well as reduce appetite and the number of calories your body absorbs from mixed meals. Berries contain the antioxidant ellagic acid which may help decrease wrinkling and other signs of skin aging related to sun exposure.

If You Like Pina Colada

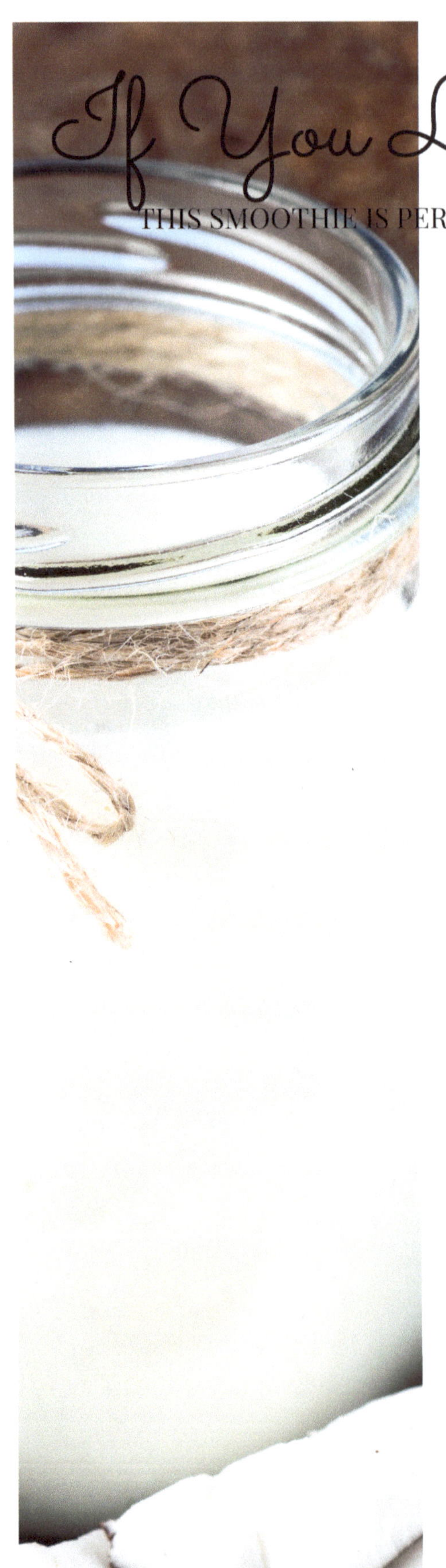

Start your Friday or any day with your favorite libation. It makes you feel just like those ones with the alcohol, or better. There's a reason this blend is desired. Don't deny yourself it's goodness.

You will need

- 1-1½ cup coconut milk
- ½ banana
- ½ cup frozen strawberries
- ½ cup frozen pineapple

Optional Ingredients

- Vanilla flavored plant based protein powder
- Sea moss

To Make

Add all ingredients to the blender. Be sure to add the powdered and liquid ingredients last to minimize the mess and maximize your blender's ability. Blend until smooth. Add more liquid for a thinner smoothie, less for a thicker smoothie.

Notes

Tired of smoothies in a cup!? Blend this mixture thick and serve in a bowl. Top with your favorite berries, nuts, seeds, whip cream, etc Switch up the Strawberries with Mango for a tropical Colada Strawberries packed with vitamins, fiber, and particularly high levels of antioxidants known as polyphenols, strawberries are sodium-free, fat-free, cholesterol-free, low-calorie food. They are among the top 20 fruits in antioxidant capacity and are a good source of manganese and potassium.

Dreamsicle

IT WAS ALL A DREAM

Who knew that these things blended up in a cup would be so delicious and nutritious. Just as sweet and delicious as the childhood favorite popsicle. Good for you and good to you! Dreams do come true.

You will need

- ½ or 1 cup unsweetened non-dairy milk
- ½ cup orange juice
- ¼ cup vanilla yogurt
- ½ cup peeled, diced sweet potatoes
- ½ banana
- ½ orange or 1 large clementine
- ½ cup sliced carrots

Optional Ingredients

- Sea moss
- Vanilla plant based protein powder

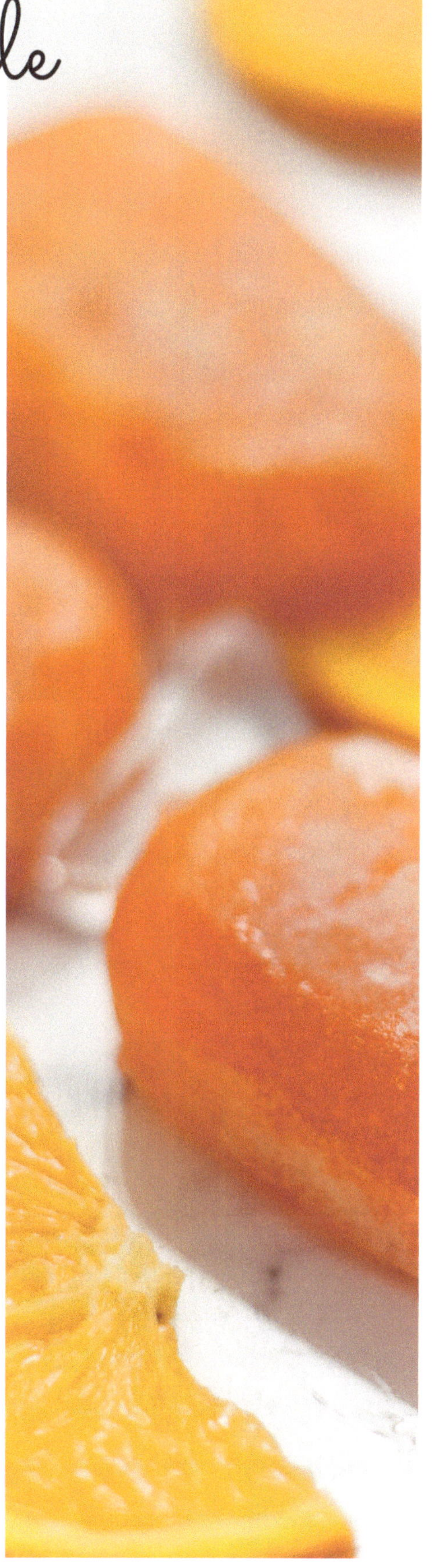

To Make

Add all ingredients to the blender. Be sure to add the powdered and liquid ingredients last to minimize the mess and maximize your blender's ability. Blend until smooth. Add more liquid for a thinner smoothie, less for a thicker smoothie.

Notes

Oranges by nature are rich in Vitamin C and fiber, providing powerful benefits to your immune system while also keeping you full and satisfied.

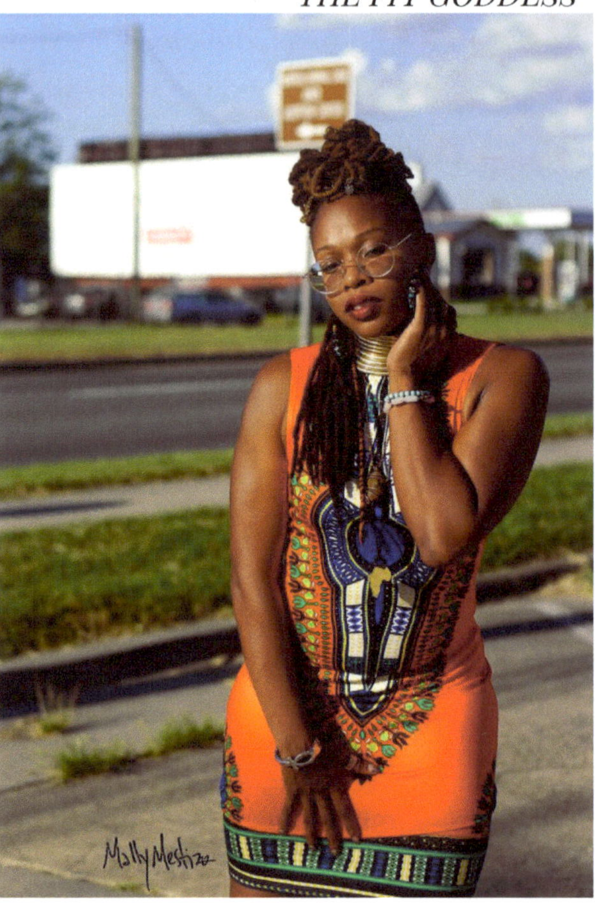

Jara Clark
THE FIT GODDESS

After children, Jara found herself heavier than she had ever been. At the time, she had been telling
her oldest son, then five years old that the three main components to a healthy life included eating, sleeping, and exercising. Soon she realized she wasn't following her own words and immediately decided to get a gym membership with her local YMCA.

After enrolling, she began trying class after class until she fell in love with Zumba. After about a year of consistency she needed more of a challenge and was introduced to the then Hip Hop Class, now called MIXXEDFIT. There she learned some harsh truths about her own self-love. Through discipline and consistency, she began to witness not only her physical form change but her mindset change.

As a graduate of Norfolk State University with a Bachelor's Degree in Psychology Jara understands that our physical strength depends on our mental agility. The two have a symbiotic relationship. Her goal is to help individuals realize that fitness is more mental than it is physical and that growth through fitness can be an all-encompassing change of mind, body, and spirit. In her practice as a personal trainer, she helps individuals achieve their weight loss goals but more importantly, to live healthy inside and out. Jara's strong love of dance caused her to get her certification to become a MIXXEDFIT instructor. She is also certified in first aid, AED, and CPR. Join the tribe! Contact her to start your journey today.

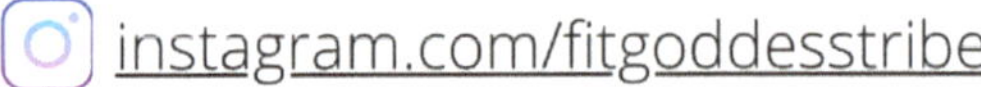 instagram.com/fitgoddesstribe   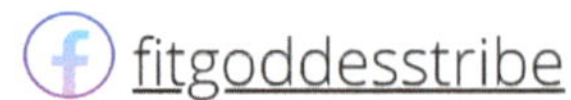 fitgoddesstribe   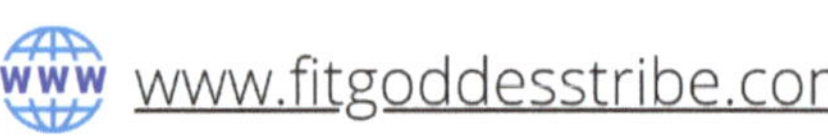 www.fitgoddesstribe.com

www.ingramcontent.com/pod-product-compliance
Lightning Source LLC
Chambersburg PA
CBHW040152240726
48664CB00002B/679